The Complete Mediterranean Diet Cookbook For Beginners

Healthy and Easy Recipes for Every Day

1st Edition

Dave P. Adams

Copyright © 2019 by Dave P. Adams

All rights reserved

All rights for this book here presented belong exclusively to the author.
Usage or reproduction of the text is forbidden and requires a clear consent of the author in case of expectations.

ISBN – 9781691838844

TABLE OF CONTENTS

INTRODUCTION 7
- **What is The Mediterranean Diet?** 8
- **The Mediterranean Diet: Getting Started** 11
  - Foods That You Should Exclude 11
  - Foods To Eat In Moderation 12
  - Foods To Eat 12

RECIPES 15
- **Breakfast Recipes** 17
  - Mediterranean Scrambled Eggs 18
  - Watermelon Pizza with Feta and Balsamic Sauce 20
  - Pizza with Avocado, Tomato, and Gouda Cheese 21
  - Keto Egg Muffins with Prosciutto 23
  - Greek Guacamole 25
  - Feta Inspired Frozen Yo 26
  - Sweet Potatoes Stuffed with Avocado-Tahini and Chickpeas ... 27
  - Refreshing Tuna Salad 29
- **Meat Recipes** 31
  - Greek Plate of Steak and Hummus 32
  - Beef and Veggie Wraps 34
  - Steak Pinwheels 35
  - Mediterranean Salad Burger 37
  - Mediterranean Kofta Beef 38
  - Mediterranean Lemony Chicken Soup 40
  - Quick Chicken Marsala 42
  - Lamb and Beet Meatballs 44
  - Zucchini-Sausage Pizza with Pesto Sauce 46
  - Mediterranean Chicken Cucumber Salad 48
  - Gyro-Inspired Turkey Burgers 50
  - Peach Chicken Salad with Bulgur 52

TABLE OF CONTENTS

Seafood Recipes ... 55
- Slow Cooked Salmon ... 56
- Grilled Striped Bass with Tomatoes and Olives ... 57
- Couscous with Tuna and Pepperoncini ... 59
- Tilapia with Parmesan and Pesto ... 61
- Cod with Swiss Chard and Orange ... 63
- Sheet-Pan Salmon with Honey Mustard ... 65
- One-Pan Baked Rosemary Citrus Salmon ... 67

Vegetable Recipes ... 69
- Sheet-Pan Roasted Vegetables ... 70
- Brown Rice and Parsley Pilaf ... 72
- Braised Fingerling Potatoes ... 74
- Honey Glazed Eggplant ... 76
- Jambalaya Vegan Style ... 78

Salad Recipes ... 81
- Easy Mediterranean Salad ... 82
- Lettuce Cups Egg Salad ... 84
- Mediterranean Salad for Everyday ... 85
- Balela Salad ... 87
- Pasta and Hummus Salad ... 89

Snacks & Dessert Recipes ... 91
- Choc Chip Cookies ... 92
- Nutty Choc Brownies ... 94
- Choc Mousse ... 96
- Quinoa Crunchies ... 97
- Glazed Peaches with hazelnuts ... 99

TIPS ON HOW TO LOSE 10 POUNDS IN TWO WEEKS WITH MEDITERRANEAN DIET 101

Eat Your Main Meal Early 102
Vegetables and Olive Oil – The Perfect Combination 102
Hydrate, Hydrate, Hydrate 102
Don't Run Away From Olive Oil 103
Walk This Day 103
Eat Right 103
Avoid The Wrong Foods 103
Stay Strict 104
Enjoy Your Food 104
Festina Lente 104

CONCLUSION 105

DISCLAIMER 107

INTRODUCTION

INTRODUCTION

Why is it that people living in the Southern regions of Spain, Italy, and Greece seem to live a longer and happier life, than those in the Western or Northern parts of Europe? The answer is that they have a unique easting lifestyle we have come to know as the Mediterranean diet. We know that for many people this answer is not a good enough explanation, but it is incredible how a healthy and balanced diet can change your life for good. Throughout this cookbook, we will take care to give you a deep insight on what the Mediterranean diet actually is, how it can be of benefit to you, and follow it all up with an array of recipes to get you started!

What is The Mediterranean Diet?

If you enjoy looking up articles that relate to health, fitness, and nutrition, you probably saw the Mediterranean diet being mentioned in a positive light. There is a good reason for it as numerous studies have shown that eating such a diet comes with a number of benefits, including reduced risks of certain diseases. To make things clear, these were not some studies that were doing research solely on the meal plans without people trying them out, on the contrary. The groups often included people that were at a high risk of cardiovascular or Alzheimer's/Parkinson's disease. What these studies concluded is that those who ate a Mediterranean diet reduced their risk by at least 30%. But why is that and how can such a meal plan benefit your health?

The idea of the Mediterranean diet dates back to 1960s when it was compared to the one that was common in the USA. That is where the above mentioned Gina Crawford quote comes from. It was quite fascinating to see that people living in a particular region were much healthier, even though they were poor and didn't have much to spend on food, unlike the wealthier people in New York. This was mostly prescribed to the low-stress lifestyle that they were living, and a diet based on eating a lot of unsaturated fat and plant-based food. The whole idea surrounding the Mediterranean diet is the opposite of what studies suggested until then, where fat was seen as the number one threat to get cardiovascular disease and, of course, obesity. Apparently, people living in Italy, France, Spain, Greece, and northern parts of Africa proved these researchers wrong. In fact, it's the sugars that should be avoided, while getting more omega 3 and omega 6 rich products should be the core of your diet. This all brings us to a realization that living by a Mediterranean meal plan means eating more plant-based foods, such as fresh fruits, vegetables, and nuts, as well as fish and eggs in moderation. As you can see, meat takes almost no part in this concept.

One of the greatest things about following the Mediterranean diet, is that it is in no-way restrictive. In fact, you will feel like you are doing cheat meals all day every day. As long as you have some time and enjoy cooking, the food common for this plan is going to become your favorite. You will get the opportunity to introduce it to other people, by cooking a nice Mediterranean plate, highlighted by, for example, ruby salmon, spinach and asparagus, some olive oil coated bread and a nice glass of red wine. The whole idea around the Mediterranean diet is to enjoy your food and eat it slowly, preferably with a group of family members or friends. As the old Latin proverb says *Festina lente,* which loosely translates to don't rush, take your time and get it right. While wine is a regular feature of this meal plan, due to it being rich in antioxidants, you should preferably make water your number one drinking priority. Staying hydrated, especially after a fibrous meal, is key to a healthy digestive tract. You should also know that food is just one part of the Mediterranean diet. The other part requires some kind of physical activity afterward. Whether it is going for a light walk, or doing some gardening, it will help you digest the food and aid other bodily functions.

The Mediterranean diet is very pretty and more colors your plate features, the better. While this diet doesn't include a lot of meat, it is in no way bland or tasteless. It ensures the perfect balance between fat, carbs, protein, and micronutrients including vitamins and minerals. Before we get into the main benefits of following this meal plan, it is important to discuss what the risks of an unhealthy diet are. From what some American studies suggest, the number one cause of obesity and premature death is a diet high in sugars and saturated fats, as well as lack of physical activity and too much stress. All this leads to an increased risk of diabetes, Alzheimer's, Parkinson's and cardiovascular problems. How do saturated fat and sugars endanger your cardiovascular health? By upping the levels of LDL while keeping the good cholesterol (high-density lipoprotein) levels low. Now that we know the root of obesity and other risks, it is much easier to address the problem and treat it with certain habit changes. With this in mind, there are more than a few benefits related to physical health that accompany the Mediterranean diet.

First of all, a diet rich in plants and fish is ideal from a holistic perspective, as it is seen to be a perfect fit for our digestive tract. People often wish to get in shape and while the Mediterranean diet doesn't revolve around weight loss, it is one of the simplest ways to do so. By cutting back on sugars and saturated fats, and eating more plants and unsaturated fats, you will increase your metabolism and limit the number of calories you eat. The reason? Whole grains, vegetables, fruits, and nuts are high in fiber, which keeps you full for a longer time, therefore decreasing your appetite, which is the absolute opposite to what sugar and simple carbs do to your body. A sugary/high carb meal results in huge energy spikes, then cravings just an hour later, so you eat again. So the first benefit of the Mediterranean diet is effective weight management and a healthier GI tract. Along with that, the type of food present in this meal plan keeps glucose levels in track, and increases the levels of the high-density lipoprotein cholesterol, more commonly known as the good cholesterol. This then reduces the chance of a potential heart attack and keeps high-blood pressure at bay. Not to forget, it is one of the best diets to do if you simple want to improve memory and general brain health. This is because of the many fresh fruit and nuts that are rich in omega 3 and omega 6 fats, which abound in this eating style. These fats are known to contribute to a better focus and memory, along with reducing chances of Alzheimer's and Parkinson's disease. Last but not least, following this food concept, along with light physical exercise, you will be more energized and effectively get on with your daily routine.

The Mediterranean region is not only beautiful to live in, due to its vivid culture, but is also great for enjoying some of the tastiest and healthiest food there is. But think about it, if you can't go and live in some of the Mediterranean countries, what you can do is bring that atmosphere home! A diet that is cheap, healthy, and tasty! It can't get much better than that! Instead of going to fancy restaurants or allowing the core of your diet to be fast-food chains, invest some time and love, and utilize all the benefits of the Mediterranean diet. Before we go ahead and introduce you to some of the great dishes that you can make at the comfort of your home, let's check out the common ingredients used and everything else that you will require, to get you started.

The Mediterranean Diet: Getting Started

Now that you have been introduced to the idea and benefits of the Mediterranean diet, we shall go ahead and give you a better insight on the foods that you should be avoiding, and those you should introduce to your meal plan. As mentioned, the whole concept is based on eating more plant-based food and fish, while cutting back on what you would usually consider essential, meat and sugars.

Foods That You Should Exclude

Starting off with foods that you should avoid, there is quite a list that you should look into. Firstly, you should be completely excluding ingredients and products that contain added sugars. We know that this sounds tough but trust us, making fresh fruit and yogurt your dessert instead of eating a sweetened candy bar is both healthier and tastier. Talking about foods with added sugars, we should also make mention of candies, ice cream, table sugar, soda, etc. There is one thing we would like to suggest, and that is that while ice cream is a no-no, homemade gelato is perfectly acceptable. It features almost no refined sugar as the main ingredients are fresh fruit, nuts, and a natural sweetener.

While bread and pasta are a common part of Italian cuisine, you should exclude them because they are made out of white flour. White flour is known to spike your glucose levels, leaving you hungry an hour after eating. As numerous studies suggest, cutting white flour out of your diet will reduce the chances of obesity, diabetes, and many other diseases connected to processed and refined ingredients. Also, margarine and processed oils should find no place in your meal plan. Completely exclude trans fats and ingredients such as soybean, canola, and cottonseed oil. Opt for extra virgin olive and coconut oil instead.

Foods such as refined meats (sausages, hot dogs) are an absolute no-no. This also goes for anything that has a low-fat label on it, as chances are that it has a high content of refined processed sugar, which is dangerous for your health.

Foods To Eat In Moderation

While the previous paragraph dealt with foods and ingredients you shouldn't eat whatsoever, there are certain dairy and meat products that you can eat but only in moderation or rarely.

Eggs are common to the Mediterranean diet, as they are a good source of protein and do contain an amount of unsaturated fat. On the other hand, they are rich in saturated fats as well, which is something you want to avoid too much of. Much like eggs, red meat is fine to eat in moderation, as it can provide you vital minerals such as zinc, selenium, and iron, but you should still focus on leafy greens and fish for the source of critical micronutrients. Poultry can be eaten more often than red meat, as long as it comes from a trusted source and is not full of antibiotics.

When it comes to dairy products, you will find cheese and yogurt to be a regular feature of the Mediterranean diet. Just remember to keep this in moderation as well, due to the high saturated fat content. Dairy is also not the perfect food to eat in combination with spinach and other greens, due to its acidic effect.

Foods To Eat

As we mentioned, the Mediterranean Diet is in no way bland or tasteless. Also, it is not that restrictive in terms of calories or sodium intake, as the whole concept lies in the quality rather than the quantity of the food that you get. However, this does not mean that you should binge, but that you don't have to stress over whether you ate more than one plate of fish and whole grains.

The core of any Mediterranean plan is whole grains as the perfect side to your salmon or tuna-based dish. There are a number of healthy grains that you can enjoy including quinoa, buckwheat, bulgur, farro, brown rice, oats, whole wheat pasta, and bread (not made with white flour!). Whether we are talking about breakfast, lunch or dinner, it is always a good idea to have some of these at your side, as these grains are rich in fiber, antioxidants, and compounds that have an anti-inflammatory effect.

Along with whole grains, the Mediterranean diet mainly uses plant-based food including fruits, vegetables, legumes, and nuts. Talking about vegetables, onions, spinach, kale, cucumbers, Brussels sprouts, and asparagus are all quite common. As for fruits, tomatoes and olives are the most common (yes these are not vegetables). Tomatoes are rich in lycopene that is critical for cardiovascular health, while olives have an abundance of omega 3 and omega 6 fats that reduce the chances of heart disease and high blood pressure. Figs, dates, melons, and peaches are also common. When it comes to nuts, walnuts, almonds, pumpkin seeds, and pine nuts are all an intrinsic part of this diet. They are rich in monosaturated fats, vitamins (A, E) and minerals. Last but not least, legumes such as beans, chickpeas, lentils, and pulses are rich in plant-based protein and are, as such, the perfect addition to this diet.

When it comes to protein sources, apart from the previously mentioned plants, you should focus on eating fish and shellfish rich in omega-3. These include sardines, tuna, salmon, mackerel and cod. Oysters and anchovies are also regularly featured on the Mediterranean plate.

Fats are an essential part of this concept, and your main source should be olive oil. Used for cooking and as a salad dressing, it is incredibly healthy and has a good balance of the omega 3 and the omega 6 fatty acids. It is connected with improved cardiovascular health, memory, and skin health.

It is no secret that red wine is a predominant feature in the Mediterranean cuisine. Whether we are talking about including it in cooking or drinking a glass as an accompanying part of the lunch/dinner routine. It is abundant in antioxidants and other compounds that could help you fight off free radicals and certain diseases. Apart from keeping the doctor away, a moderate glass of red wine will help you cope with stress and relax after hard working hours.

RECIPES

RECIPES

The idea of the Mediterranean diet is clear, and so are the foods and ingredients that you should or shouldn't include. We are now all set and ready to go ahead and explore the interesting and tasty ideas that will highlight your meal plan including breakfast, dinner, lunch and dessert dishes.

BREAKFAST RECIPES

BREAKFAST RECIPES

MEDITERRANEAN SCRAMBLED EGGS

Time: 15 minutes | Serves: 2
Net Carbs: 13 g | Fiber: 3 g | Protein: 14 g
Fat: 17 g | Kcal (per serving): 249

INGREDIENTS:

- 4 eggs
- 1 yellow-pepper, diced
- 2 sliced spring onions
- 8 quartered cherry tomatoes
- 2 tablespoon of sliced olives
- 1 tablespoon of capers
- 1 tablespoon of olive oil
- ¼ teaspoon of dried oregano
- Black pepper
- Fresh parsley

PREPARATION:

1. Start by heating one tablespoon of olive oil in a skillet and adding the diced yellow pepper and sliced onions. Stew these for a few minutes, only to then add tomatoes, capers, and olives. Continue to cooking on a medium heat for one minute.

2. Once the vegetables are ready, crack your eggs and scramble them into the veg. Cook for a few minutes, stirring the eggs constantly, to achieve the velvety texture. While you are doing that, add the black pepper and oregano, and should you want to, a pinch of salt.

3. Now that your scrambled eggs with veggies are ready, serve them on a plate and top it off with some fresh chopped parsley.

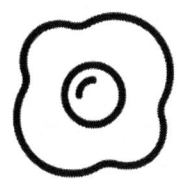

WATERMELON PIZZA WITH FETA AND BALSAMIC SAUCE

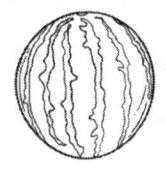

Time: 15 minutes | Serves: 4
Net Carbs: 14 g | Fiber: 1 g | Protein: 2 g
Fat: 3 g | Kcal (per serving): 90

INGREDIENTS:

- 1 watermelon slice
- 1 oz./28 g Feta cheese
- 6 olives (Kalamata)
- 1 tsp fresh mint leaves
- ½ tablespoons balsamic sauce

PREPARATION:

1. You should start by slicing a watermelon in half. From one half, take a 1" thick slice and lay it flat. Slice this piece into "pizza triangles" and this will be your pizza base.

2. You will need a round pan/plate that is usually used for baking pizza, on which you will put the watermelon wedges (pizza slices), arranging them in a circular fashion. Start by covering those wedges in feta cheese, and add olives next. Top it all off with balsamic sauce and fresh mint leaves. Voila, you are set and good to go as this recipe requires no baking or grilling!

PIZZA WITH AVOCADO, TOMATO, AND GOUDA CHEESE

Time: 40 minutes | Serves: 4
Net Carbs: 37 g | Fiber: 10 g | Protein: 15g
Fat: 25 g | Kcal (per serving): 416

INGREDIENTS:

- **For Crust**
- 1 cup chickpea flour
- 1 cup cold water
- 2 tablespoons olive oil
- ¼ teaspoons sea salt
- ¼ teaspoon black pepper
- 1 teaspoon minced garlic
- 1 teaspoon onion powder

For Toppings

- 1 sliced Roma tomato
- Half of an avocado
- 2 oz./28 g thinly sliced Gouda cheese
- ⅓ cup tomato sauce
- 3 tablespoons green onions
- Extra pepper, red flakes to top

PIZZA WITH AVOCADO, TOMATO, AND GOUDA CHEESE

PREPARATION:

1. Mix all the ingredients for the crust, until you get a batter like texture. Whisk either using a fork or using a hand mixer until the batter is smooth. Once that is done, let the batter sit for around 20 minutes at regular room temperature. While you are waiting for it to rest, preheat the pan in an oven at 425 degrees F/220 degrees Celsius (10 minutes).

2. Prepare your vegetables needed for the topping. Carefully take out the pan out the oven, and put it aside. Coat the pan in olive oil and then pour in the chickpea batter. Tilt the pan as much as you need until it is completely covered in the batter. Once that is set, put the pan back in the oven for another 8 minutes at the same temperature.

3. Take the crust out the oven and add the tomato sauce and vegetables. Ensure you spread the tomato sauce over the baked crust, and continue by putting tomatoes and avocado on top. After that, you should sprinkle thinly sliced Gouda cheese, green onions and a little drizzle of olive oil. Continue baking for about 15 minutes or until the crust is brown and crispy.

4. Take the pan out of the oven. Allow to cool for 5 minutes. Sprinkle some more pepper and red flakes on top and serve.

KETO EGG MUFFINS WITH PROSCIUTTO

Time: 25 minutes | Serves: 6
Net Carbs: 2 g | Fiber: 2 g | Protein: 9g
Fat: 6 g | Kcal (per serving): 109

INGREDIENTS:

- 9 Slices Prosciutto
- ½ cup of canned roasted red pepper, sliced + additional for garnish
- ⅓ cup of fresh spinach, minced
- ¼ cup of feta cheese, crumbled
- 5 large eggs
- A pinch of salt
- A pinch of pepper
- 1 ½ tablespoons of Pesto sauce
- Some fresh basil for garnish

KETO EGG MUFFINS WITH PROSCIUTTO

PREPARATION:

1. Preheat your oven to 400°F/200°C, and coating the muffin tin using a non-stick cooking spray. Cover the base of each muffin spot with one and a half slice of Prosciutto, and continue by placing roasted red pepper over it (not too much). Once you have done that it is time to top it all off with ½ tablespoon of feta cheese.

2. In a medium bowl, whisk the eggs together with the salt and pepper. Make sure that the mixture is smooth and easily divided. Pour the same amount in each muffin tin.

3. Bake for 15 minutes, or until you can see that the eggs are set. Once it is baked, remove the muffin and use the parsley and a bit more roasted red paper for garnishing.

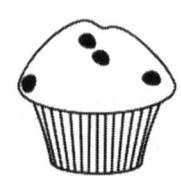

GREEK GUACAMOLE

Time: 10 minutes | Serves: 8
Net Carbs: 6 g | Fiber: 4 g | Protein: 1 g
Fat: 10 g | Kcal (per serving): 110

INGREDIENTS:

- 2 large ripe avocados (halved, pit removed)
- 2 tablespoons of lemon juice
- 1 heaped tablespoon of chopped sun-dried tomatoes
- 3 tablespoons of diced cherry tomatoes
- ¼ cup of diced red onion
- 1 teaspoons of dried oregano
- 2 tablespoons of fresh chopped parsley
- 4 whole kalamata olives (pitted and chopped)
- 1 pinch each of sea salt and black pepper

PREPARATION:

1. In a medium bowl, add the avocado and lemon juice together, using a potato masher or a fork. Once you have done that, it is time to add remaining the ingredients including tomatoes and olives. Add spices to suit your preference.

2. For added acidity, add some more lemon juice, or alternatively, for some kick, add some parsley or oregano. For a deeper flavor, leave it in the fridge overnight. Add some parsley for garnish, just before serving.

FETA INSPIRED FROZEN YO

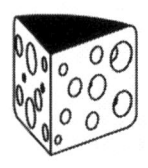

Time: 5 minutes | Serves: 3
Net Carbs: 7 g | Fiber: 0 g | Protein: 7 g
Fat: 10 g | Kcal (per serving): 161

INGREDIENTS:

- 1 cup of plain Greek yogurt
- ½ cup of feta cheese
- 1 tablespoons honey

PREPARATION:

1. Put all the ingredients in a wide bowl and mix until it all combines.
2. Pour it in a food processor and let it run until you achieve a smooth texture. After that, return it to the wide bowl, and put it in a freezer.
3. Freeze until the mixture becomes solid.
4. Break it into cubes and return it to blender. Try to achieve a creamy, yogurt-like consistency. You can add some water or milk to aid you in the process. Serve immediately with a drizzle of honey on top.

Time: 50 minutes | Serves: 8
Net Carbs: 38 g | Fiber: 8 g | Protein: 7 g
Fat: 15 g | Kcal (per serving): 308

INGREDIENTS:

- 8 medium-sized potatoes

Marinated Chickpeas

- 15oz./420 g can of chickpeas, drained and rinsed
- ½ a red pepper, diced
- 3 tablespoons of extra virgin olive oil
- 1 tablespoon of fresh lemon juice
- 1 tablespoon of lemon zest
- 1 clove of garlic, crushed
- 1 tablespoon of freshly chopped parsley
- 1 tablespoon of fresh oregano
- ¼ teaspoon of sea salt

Avocado-Tahini Sauce

- 1 medium-sized ripe avocado
- ¼ cup of tahini
- ¼ cup water
- 1 clove of garlic, crushed
- 1 tablespoon of fresh parsley
- 1 tablespoon of fresh lemon juice

Toppings:

- ¼ cup of pepitas
- Crumbled up vegan feta (for the dairy free version)

SWEET POTATOES STUFFED WITH AVOCADO-TAHINI AND CHICKPEAS

PREPARATION:

1. Preheat the oven to 400°F/200°C. Place all the potatoes on a baking tray and pierce a few holes through each, in order to prevent the air from staying trapped.
2. Bake for about an hour until the potatoes are tender and brown.
3. Combine the chickpeas with the ingredients for the marinade and let it sit for 45 minutes.
4. For the avocado-tahini sauce, add all the ingredients to a blender and process until you achieve a smooth consistency. If it seems too thick, simply add more water.
5. Once the potatoes are out, let them cool down for 10 minutes. Then slit the potatoes down the middle and spoon the marinated chickpeas in. Top it all off with the avocado-tahini sauce, and serve immediately.

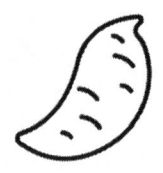

Time: 8 minutes | Serves: 2
Net Carbs: 3 g | Fiber: 1 g | Protein: 21 g
Fat: 17 g | Kcal (per serving): 250

REFRESHING TUNA SALAD

INGREDIENTS:

- 10oz./280 g of drained Tuna
- 2 tablespoons of capers
- 8 sliced of Kalamata olives
- ¼ cup of diced red peppers
- 1 tablespoons of lemon juice
- 2tablespoons of olive oil
- Salt and pepper to taste

PREPARATION:

1. Combine all the ingredients in a medium bowl, and whisk with a fork, until all is well combined.
2. You can serve it over a muffin or lettuce immediately, or after a few hours left in the fridge.

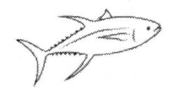

MEAT RECIPES

MEAT RECIPES

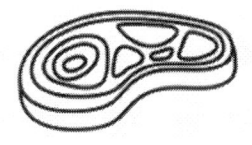

GREEK PLATE OF STEAK AND HUMMUS

Time: 30 minutes | Serves: 4
Net Carbs: 19 g | Fiber: 8 g | Protein: 33 g
Fat: 18 g | Kcal (per serving): 372

INGREDIENTS:

- 1 lb/1 kg of beef (Top Sirloin Steaks Boneless, cut 1 inch thick)
- 1 medium cucumber
- 3 tablespoons of fresh lemon juice
- ¼ teaspoon of pepper
- 1 cup of ready-to-serve hummus
- Romesco sauce

Rub:

- ¼ cup oregano leaves (chopped)
- 1 tablespoon of grated lemon peel
- 1 tablespoon of garlic
- 1 teaspoon of pepper

PREPARATION:

1. Start by mixing the rub ingredients together and pressing them into the sliced beef tenderloin.
2. Place your steaks on a grill, letting them sit there from 10 to 17 minutes depending on how you like your beef done (turn occasionally).
3. Slice and prepare the cucumber by mixing it with the lemon juice and pepper.
4. Once the steaks are done, carve them into slices and sprinkle some salt and pepper to taste.
5. Serve with ¼ cup of hummus on each side, and Romesco sauce drizzled on top of the beef.
6. Garnish with sliced cucumber, pita chips, or olives.

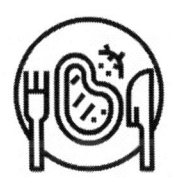

BEEF AND VEGGIE WRAPS

Time: 5 minutes | Serves: 4
Net Carbs: 31 g | Fiber: 4 g | Protein: 22 g
Fat: 8 g | Kcal (per serving): 290

INGREDIENTS:

- 12 oz./ 336 g sliced cooked beef (steak)
- 4 whole wheat flour tortillas
- Hummus
- Peppers, carrots, tomatoes (to taste)
- Spinach, arugula (to taste)

PREPARATION:

1. Cover a skillet with a non-stick cooking spray. Heat the whole wheat tortillas over medium temperature for about one minute on each side.
2. Spread hummus evenly leaving about ¼ inch uncovered around the edges.
3. Mix the vegetables and greens and add on top of the hummus.
4. Top it all off with sliced beef and roll firmly.

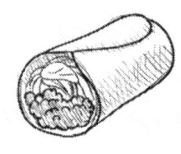

STEAK PINWHEELS

Time: 15minutes | Serves: 5
Net Carbs: 8 g | Fiber: 2 g | Protein: 27 g
Fat: 13 g | Kcal (per serving): 117

INGREDIENTS:

- 1 lb./ 450 g beef steak
- ⅓ cup of lemon juice
- 2 tablespoons of olive oil
- 2 tablespoons of dried oregano leaves
- ⅓ cup of olive tapenade
- ¼ cup of crumbled feta cheese
- 1 cup of frozen spinach
- 4 cups of cherry tomatoes
- Salt to taste

STEAK PINWHEELS

PREPARATION:

1. Cover the beef in plastic wrap and pound it up to around ½ inches of thickness. Remove from plastic.
2. Mix olive oil, dried oregano leaves and lemon juice as marinade ingredients, and coat both sides of the flank. Leave it in a bag to refrigerate for around 4 hours.
3. Preheat the oven to 425°F/220°C
4. Placing baking paper over a baking sheet.
5. Take out your steak and place it on a cutting board. Spread the tapenade and top it off with spinach and feta.
6. Roll the steak into a log and tie it up using kitchen strings. Slice it into six even pieces, and pour the remains of the marinade over it. Arrange tomatoes around the beef pinwheels.
7. Roast for around 30 minutes or until tender
8. Allow to cool for 5 minutes.

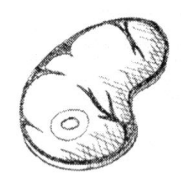

MEDITERRANEAN SALAD BURGER

Time: 25 minutes | Serves: 4
Net Carbs: 16 g | Fiber: 3 g | Protein: 29 g
Fat: 10 g | Kcal (per serving): 267

INGREDIENTS:

- 4 cooked Ground beef burgers (3 oz./75 g)
- 2 cups of chopped cucumber
- 2 cups of Romaine lettuce
- 2 cups of chopped tomatoes
- ½ cup of diced red onion
- ½ cup of reduced fat Greek-dressing
- ¼ cup of crumbled feta cheese
- 2 tablespoons of Kalamata olives

PREPARATION:

1. Microwave the burgers for about 2 minutes.
2. Combine the vegetables in a medium bowl, and toss them around with the Greek dressing.
3. Divide the vegetable mixture onto four plates.
4. Place the burger on top of the lettuce mixture and top it off with some Kalamata olives and crumbled Feta cheese. Serve immediately.

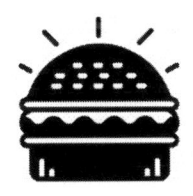

MEDITERRANEAN KOFTA BEEF

Time: 25 minutes | Serves: 4
Net Carbs: 2 g | Fiber: 1 g | Protein: 22 g
Fat: 12 g | Kcal (per serving): 216

INGREDIENTS:

- 1 pound/453 g Ground Beef (93% lean or leaner)
- ½ cup of diced onions
- 1 tablespoon of olive oil
- ½ teaspoon of salt
- ½ teaspoon of ground coriander
- ½ teaspoon of ground cumin
- ¼ teaspoon of ground cinnamon
- ¼ teaspoon of all-spice
- ¼ teaspoon of dried mint leaves

PREPARATION:

1. In a large bowl, combine the beef, onion, salt, coriander, cumin, cinnamon, all-spice and mint leaves. Mix gently, but thoroughly.
2. Taking a quarter of the beef mixture, shape is around 8" skewers. Be sure to leave about 1" or 2" at the bottom of the skewer.
3. With your fingers, make small dents along the beef kofta, about 1" apart.
4. Continue this process with the rest of the kofta mixture and 3 skewers.
5. Chill in the fridge for a minimum of 10 minutes.
6. Grill the koftas in the center of a warm grill. Try to avoid turning them too soon, as they could break. Grill for 12 – 14 minutes, or until cooked through.

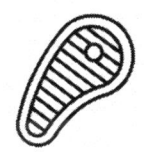

MEDITERRANEAN LEMONY CHICKEN SOUP

Time: 20 minutes | Serves: 6
Net Carbs: 16 g | Fiber: 3 g | Protein: 32 g
Fat: 8 g | Kcal (per serving): 261

INGREDIENTS:

- 1 tablespoon of olive oil
- 3/4 cup of carrot, cubed
- ½ cup of chopped yellow onion
- 2 teaspoons minced fresh garlic
- ¾ teaspoon of crushed red pepper
- 6 cups unsalted chicken stock
- ½ cup of uncooked whole-wheat orzo
- 3 large eggs
- ¼ cup of fresh lemon juice
- 3 cups of shredded rotisserie chicken
- 3 cups of chopped baby spinach
- 1 ¼ teaspoons of kosher salt
- ½ teaspoon of black pepper
- 3 tablespoons of chopped fresh dill

PREPARATION:

1. Prepare a Dutch oven by lightly coating it with extra virgin olive oil. Heat it to a medium temperature and start cooking onions and carrots together for about 3 to 4 minutes. Once carrots and onions have softened, add garlic and red pepper. Continue stirring for a couple of minutes.
2. Add stock to the pot and bring everything to boiling. Add whole wheat orzo and cook it together until it is al dente.
3. Whisk the eggs and the lemon juice together in a medium bowl, gradually adding stock while you are mixing.
4. Lower the heat to low and mix in egg-lemon juice mixture, chicken, spinach, salt and the pepper into the pot. Cook for a few minutes more or until spinach wilts.
5. Divide the soup into six separate bowls and sprinkle some fresh dill on top.

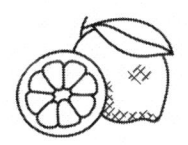

QUICK CHICKEN MARSALA

Time: 20 minutes | Serves: 4
Net Carbs: 9 g | Fiber: 1 g | Protein: 28 g
Fat: 17 g | Kcal (per serving): 344

INGREDIENTS:

- 2 tablespoons of olive oil, divided between 2 separate tablespoons
- 4 skinless, boneless chicken breast cutlets
- ¾ teaspoon of black pepper, divided into ¼ and ½ teaspoons
- ½ teaspoon of kosher salt, divided into ¼'s
- 10 oz./280 g. pre-sliced button mushrooms
- 4 thyme sprigs
- 1 tablespoon of all-purpose flour
- 2/3 cup of unsalted chicken stock
- 2/3 cup of Marsala wine
- 2 ½ tablespoons of unsalted butter
- 1 tablespoon of chopped fresh thyme

PREPARATION:

1. Heat one of your tablespoons of olive oil in a non-stick pan.
2. Season your chicken breast cutlets with the ¼ teaspoon of salt and ½ teaspoon of pepper.
3. Cook for 4 minutes per side, until the chicken is golden brown.
4. Once the chicken is done remove it from the pan without wiping the oils and the juice that chicken has released.
5. To the same pan, add another tablespoon of olive oil, mushrooms, and thyme sprigs. Cook for around 6 minutes until browned.
6. Add flour and continue stirring for a minute more.
7. Add the wine and stock to the pan, bringing everything to boiling.
8. Add the remaining spices, and bring the chicken back to the pan. Cook for a few more minutes, and remove the sprigs just before the end. Serve with pita as a side.

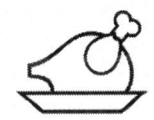

LAMB AND BEET MEATBALLS

Time: 20 minutes | Serves: 4
Net Carbs: 25 g | Fiber: 5 g | Protein: 14 g
Fat: 21 g | Kcal (per serving): 338

INGREDIENTS:

- 10 oz./280 g vacuum-packed cooked beets (such as Love Beets)
- ½ cup of uncooked bulgur
- 1 teaspoon of ground cumin
- ¾ teaspoon of kosher salt, divided into ½ and ¼ teaspoons
- ¾ teaspoon of freshly ground black pepper
- 6oz./168 g of ground lamb
- ⅓ cup of almond flour
- 1 tablespoon of olive oil
- ½ cup of grated cucumber
- ½ cup of reduced-fat sour-cream
- 2 tablespoons of thinly sliced fresh mint
- 2 tablespoons of fresh lemon juice
- 4 cups mixed baby greens

PREPARATION:

1. Start by preheating the oven to 425°F/204°C.
2. In a blender, process the beets until they are finely chopped.
3. Combine the lamb meat, beets, cumin, bulgur, salt, pepper and almond flour in a large bowl. Go for 12 smaller meatballs.
4. Once meatballs have been shaped, cook them in a non-stick skillet for about 4 minutes or until you see a nice brown coating.
5. Place the whole pan, with the meatballs, in the preheated oven and bake for around 8 minutes.
6. In another mixing bowl, combine cucumber, sour cream, lemon juice, sea salt and mint to make a light dressing.
7. Take the pan out of the oven and serve the meatballs on four plates. Top it all off with the dressing and use greens for side garnishing.

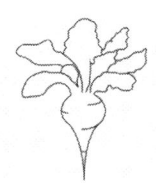

ZUCCHINI-SAUSAGE PIZZA WITH PESTO SAUCE

Time: 20 minutes | Serves: 4
Net Carbs: 44 g | Fiber: 6 g | Protein: 15 g
Fat: 22 g | Kcal (per serving): 392

INGREDIENTS:

- 3 oz./75 g ground mild Italian turkey sausage
- 1 cup thinly sliced zucchini
- 4 tablespoons of refrigerated basil pesto, divided into 1 and 3 tablespoons
- 1 pkg. of 3 (7-inch) prebaked pizza crusts (such as Mama Marys)
- 3 oz./75 g fresh, thinly sliced mozzarella cheese
- ⅛ teaspoon of crushed red pepper
- 2 tablespoons of fresh basil leaves

PREPARATION:

1. Heat a non-stick skillet on a medium-high temperature and add the ground sausage to it. Cook for around 5 minutes, breaking the sausage in the process using a spoon or a fork. Once it is cooked, remove it from the pan, without wiping the oil or juice.

2. Add the zucchini and a tablespoon of pesto sauce to the same pan, cooking for about 3 minutes.

3. Preheat your oven to 450°F/220°C.

4. Place the pizza crusts on a baking sheet and use the remaining pesto sauce (3 tablespoons) to cover the base.

5. Top the crust with the zucchini mixture, sausages, red pepper, and some crumbled mozzarella.

6. Bake for around 6-8 minutes and remove from the oven. Add a finishing touch by sprinkling some basil leaves and a little bit more of mozzarella.

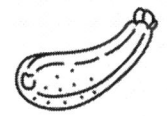

MEDITERRANEAN CHICKEN CUCUMBER SALAD

Time: 15 minutes | Serves: 6
Net Carbs: 26 g | Fiber: 7 g | Protein: 40 g
Fat: 26 g | Kcal (per serving): 482

INGREDIENTS:

- 2 cups of packed fresh flat-leaf parsley leaves (from 1 bunch)
- 1 cup of fresh baby spinach
- 2 tablespoons of fresh lemon juice
- 1 tablespoon of toasted pine nuts
- 1 tablespoon of grated Parmesan cheese
- 1 medium garlic clove, smashed
- 1 teaspoon of kosher salt
- ¼ teaspoon of black pepper
- ½ cup of extra-virgin olive oil
- 4 cups of shredded rotisserie chicken
- 2 cups of cooked, shelled edamame
- 15 oz./420 g can of unsalted chickpeas, drained and rinsed
- 1 cup of chopped English cucumber
- 4 cups of arugula

PREPARATION:

1. Start by putting the pine nuts, lemon juice, spinach, parsley, cheese, garlic, salt and pepper in a blender for about a minute.
2. Add a bit of olive oil and blend for another minute.
3. Take a large bowl and combine chickpeas, edamame, cucumber, and chicken together. Toss around and add an amount of pesto sauce.
4. Separate into six bowls, and top each off with a 2/3 cup of arugula and a cup of the dressing.

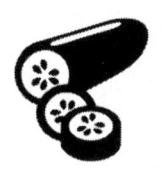

GYRO-INSPIRED TURKEY BURGERS

Time: 20 minutes | Serves: 4
Net Carbs: 28 g | Fiber: 4 g | Protein: 22 g
Fat: 17 g | Kcal (per serving): 375

INGREDIENTS:

- 1 lb./453 g 93% of lean ground turkey
- ¼ cup of canola mayonnaise
- 2 teaspoons of dried oregano
- 1 teaspoon of ground cumin
- ¼ teaspoon of kosher salt
- ¼ teaspoon black pepper, divided into two ⅛ teaspoons
- Cooking spray
- ⅓ cup plain of whole-milk Greek yogurt
- ⅓ cup of chopped kalamata olives
- 1 tablespoon of fresh lemon juice
- 4 whole-wheat hamburger buns
- 2 cups of arugula
- ½ cup of sliced cucumber
- ½ cup of thinly sliced red onion

PREPARATION:

1. Combine turkey, cumin, mayo, oregano, ⅛ teaspoon pepper, and salt and make 4 medium patties.

2. Place a non-stick skillet on a medium-high temperature and coat with a tablespoon of olive oil. Cook each burger for around 5 minutes per side, until they are golden brown.

3. Combine yogurt, olives, lemon juice, salt and the last ⅛ teaspoon of pepper in a bowl to make a dressing. Spread it over both the top and bottom of the bun. Follow up by placing arugula, the cooked burger, red onion, and cucumber.

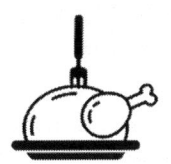

PEACH CHICKEN SALAD WITH BULGUR

Time: 20 minutes | Serves: 4
Net Carbs: 30 g | Fiber: 6 g | Protein: 31 g
Fat: 14 g | Kcal (per serving): 364

INGREDIENTS:

- 1⅓ cups of water
- ⅔ cup of bulgur
- Cooking spray
- 1 pound of chicken breast cutlets
- 1 teaspoon kosher salt, divided into two ½ teaspoons
- ½ teaspoon of black pepper
- 4 cups of packed arugula
- 2 cups of halved cherry tomatoes
- 2 cups of sliced fresh peaches
- 3 tablespoons of extra-virgin olive oil
- 2 tablespoons of rice vinegar

PREPARATION:

1. Bring the water and bulgur to a boil. Cook for around 10 minutes until it is al dente. Drain the bulgur and set aside.
2. Season the chicken cutlets in with ½ teaspoon of salt and the pepper.
3. Coat a non-stick skillet in the olive oil and cook the chicken for around 7 minutes, on a medium-high temperature, turning occasionally.
4. Let it rest for around 3 minutes, and then cut it into thin strips.
5. Combine the cooked bulgur with the arugula, tomatoes, peaches, adding vinegar and the remaining ½ teaspoon of salt.
6. Top off the chicken with the bulgur mixture and serve.

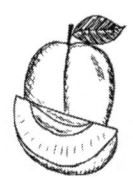

SEAFOOD RECIPES

SEAFOOD RECIPES

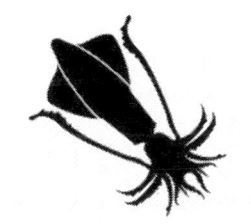

SLOW COOKED SALMON

Time: 25 minutes | Serves: 2
Net Carbs: 3.54 g | Fiber: 1.1 g | Protein: 22.99 g
Fat: 14.33 g | Kcal (per serving): 230

INGREDIENTS:

- 2 6oz salmon filets with their skin on
- A pinch Kosher salt
- 1 teaspoon crushed black pepper
- 1 teaspoon smoke paprika
- ½ teaspoon lightly crushed fennel seeds
- 1 lemon, completely zested and then halved
- ¼ cup freshly chopped dill
- 3 tablespoons extra-virgin olive oil

PREPARATION:

1. Take each salmon filet and season with the salt, pepper, and half the paprika, half of the fennel seeds, half of the lemon zest and half of the dill.
2. Using a large skillet, pour in your olive oil and add the filets. Heat on the lowest setting and allow the filets to cook for about 20 to 25 minutes, undisturbed. The top of the salmon will be bright pink, and the sides will be completely opaque. The filet should be firm to the touch.
3. Using a spatula, carefully remove the salmon from the skillet, and place on paper towels to drain off any excess oil.
4. Transfer to dinner plates, garnish with the remaining paprika, fennel seeds, lemon zest and dill and enjoy!

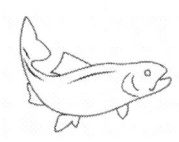

GRILLED STRIPED BASS WITH TOMATOES AND OLIVES

Time: 20 minutes | Serves: 4
Net Carbs: 21.13 g | Fiber: 12.6 g | Protein: 40.72 g
Fat: 39.01 g | Kcal (per serving): 592

INGREDIENTS:

- 4 6oz striped bass filets with their skin on (can opt for grouper, mahi mahi or halibut, if desired)
- ½ teaspoon of salt
- 1 teaspoon herbs de provence
- 1 tablespoon Dijon mustard
- 3 diced medium-sized tomatoes
- ⅓ cup of mixed pitted olives, chopped roughly
- 1 tablespoon of capers
- 1 minced garlic clove
- 2 tablespoons olive oil
- 1 tablespoon white wine vinegar
- Optional garnish: chopped mixed herbs (parsley, thyme, chives, etc)

PREPARATION:

1. Preheat your broiler/griller.
2. In cold water, rinse the fish filets and dry with a paper towel. Place the filets on a baking sheet or in an oven-proof skillet. Season the fish with the salt and the herbs. Lavishly coat the tops of your fish with the Dijon mustard.
3. In a medium mixing bowl, combine the tomatoes, capers, garlic, olives, olive oil, vinegar and ½ teaspoon salt. Once all mixed together, drizzle over the fish filets.
4. Under the broiler/griller, bake the filets for 10 minutes. After 5 minutes, rotate the pan to ensure equal browning.
5. Garnish with herbs if you so desire, and serve.

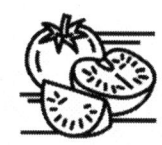

COUSCOUS WITH TUNA AND PEPPERONCINI

Time: 15 minutes | Serves: 4
Net Carbs: 14.87 g | Fiber: 1.6 g | Protein: 33.61 g
Fat: 7.44 g | Kcal (per serving): 261

INGREDIENTS:

- 1 cup chicken broth or water
- 1¼ cups couscous
- ¾ teaspoon kosher salt
- 2 5oz cans of tuna in oil
- 1 pint cherry tomatoes, chopped in half
- ½ cup of sliced pepperoncini
- ⅓ cup mixed chopped parsley
- ¼ cup of capers
- A drizzle of extra-virgin olive oil
- Kosher salt
- Black pepper, freshly ground
- 1 quartered lemon

COUSCOUS WITH TUNA AND PEPPERONCINI

PREPARATION:

1. Pour your chicken broth or water into a small cooking pot and over a medium heat, bring it to a boil.
2. Take the pot from the heat and mix the couscous well.
3. Cover the pot and let it rest for 10 minutes.
4. In a medium bowl, add the tuna, chopped cherry tomatoes, pepperoncini, capers and the parsley and combine.
5. Using a fork, fluff up your couscous, season it with a little salt and pepper, and drizzle with some olive oil.
6. Add the tuna mixture on the couscous and serve along with the lemon wedges.

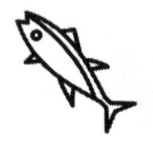

TILAPIA WITH PARMESAN AND PESTO

Time: 15 minutes | Serves: 4
Net Carbs: 4.38 g | Fiber: 0.6 g | Protein: 38.35 g
Fat: 10.31 g | Kcal (per serving): 262

INGREDIENTS:

- 4 6oz of tilapia filets
- ¼ cup of basil pesto
- ½ cup of Parmesan cheese, freshly grated
- 1 cup fresh tomatoes, chopped
- 1 teaspoon salt
- 1 teaspoon pepper
- 1 teaspoon of lemon juice
- 4 teaspoons melted butter

TILAPIA WITH PARMESAN AND PESTO

PREPARATION:

1. Preheat your broiler/griller.
2. Rinse the fish well and with a paper towel, pat it dry.
3. Cover a baking sheet with some foil and coat the foil with cooking spray or olive oil to prevent sticking.
4. Place the washed filets on the coated baking sheet.
5. On each filet, sprinkle 2 tablespoons of Parmesan cheese.
6. Broil/grill for 10 – 11 minutes, until you can see the fish is opaque and cheese is browned
7. On each piece of fish, place the fresh tomatoes and a tablespoon of the pesto.
8. Season all the filets with the salt, pepper, lemon juice and melted butter.

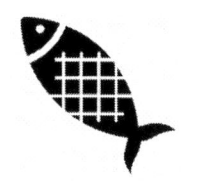

COD WITH SWISS CHARD AND ORANGE

Time: 30 minutes | Serves: 4
Net Carbs: 56.49 g | Fiber: 15 g | Protein: 44.36 g
Fat: 37.21 g | Kcal (per serving): 733

INGREDIENTS:

- 4 6oz cod filets
- 1 cup all purpose flour
- ½ teaspoon cayenne pepper
- 4 tablespoons extra virgin olive oil
- 1 teaspoon salt
- 1 teaspoon pepper
- 1 sliced red onion
- 1 orange, halved and sliced thinly
- ¼ cup fresh parsley, chopped. (Hold some extra for garnish)
- 2½ cup of Swiss chard, chopped
- 1 Orange, cut into wedges for serving

COD WITH SWISS CHARD AND ORANGE

PREPARATION:

1. On both sides of each cod fillet, season with the salt and pepper.
2. In a large bowl, combine flour and cayenne pepper.
3. Drag each piece of filet through the flour and cayenne pepper, until completely coated.
4. Heat olive oil in a large sauté pan, over a medium heat.
5. Add the cod to the heated olive oil and pan fry until browned. Should be about 3 –4 minutes on each side.
6. Remove the filets from the pan and drain the oil until you're left with about 1 tablespoon of oil in the pan.
7. Add onion and orange to the oil and sauté for about 4 – 5 minutes until onion is soft.
8. Now add the parsley and Swiss chard, and cook for 3– 4 minutes until tender.
9. Place the filets onto dinner plates and divide the Swiss charge/orange mixture between each piece of fish.
10. Garnish with more parsley and the orange wedges and serve.

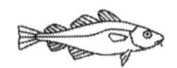

SHEET-PAN SALMON WITH HONEY MUSTARD

Time: 45 minutes | Serves: 5
Net Carbs: 28.09 g | Fiber: 5.5 g | Protein: 41.47 g
Fat: 19.14 g | Kcal (per serving): 443

INGREDIENTS:

- 1 2lbs (two pound) salmon filet
- 1 tablespoon raw honey, light in color
- 1 tablespoon coarse-grain mustard
- ½ teaspoon white wine vinegar
- 1 teaspoon salt
- 1 teaspoon pepper
- 2½ cups butternut squash, peeled, seeded and cubed
- 12 oz Brussels sprouts, halved and trimmed
- 2 cups cherry tomatoes
- 2 tablespoons avocado oil (or melted ghee)
- ½ teaspoon lemon juice, preferably freshly squeezed
- ¼ teaspoon garlic powder
- ¼ teaspoon onion powder
- ¾ teaspoon dried oregano (divided into ½ teaspoon and ¼ teaspoon)
- ⅛ teaspoon ground turmeric
- 1 thinly sliced lemon

PREPARATION:

1. Preheat oven to 400°F / 200°C.
2. Using a small mixing bowl, whisk together the honey, mustard, vinegar, the ½ teaspoon of oregano, ½ teaspoon of salt, and ¼ teaspoon of pepper.
3. Put your salmon filet into a baking dish and cover with your honey mustard marinade. Let it marinade for 15 minutes.
4. In a large bowl, combine your butternut squash cubes, Brussels sprouts, cherry tomatoes, remaining oregano, turmeric, ¼ teaspoon salt, ⅛ teaspoon pepper. Once lightly combined, toss around the edges of a large roasting pan.
5. Remove the salmon from your marinade. Allow all the excess marinade to drip off into the baking dish.
6. Put the salmon in the middle of all the vegetables and place the lemon slices along the top of the salmon.
7. Place the salmon in the oven.
8. Brush the fish with the remaining marinade, every 5 minutes.
9. Roast until the center of the fish is flaky and the veggies are crisp and soft, around 16 – 18 minutes.

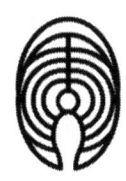

ONE-PAN BAKED ROSEMARY CITRUS SALMON

Time: 20 minutes | Serves: 3
Net Carbs: 56.49 g | Fiber: 15 g | Protein: 44.36 g
Fat: 37.21 g | Kcal (per serving): 733

INGREDIENTS:

- 3 4oz (four ounce) sockeye salmon filets
- ⅓ cup olive oil
- 1 teaspoon ground pepper
- 1 tablespoons of orange juice
- 2 tablespoons of fresh rosemary
- 2 sprigs of rosemary
- 1 tablespoon lemon juice
- ½ teaspoon minced garlic
- ¼ teaspoon of grated and dried orange peel, divided into two (ie: 2 x ⅛)
- 1 teaspoon of salt
- ¼ teaspoon of lemon pepper (optional)
- 1 bunch of thin, trimmer asparagus (or a veg of your choosing)
- 1 thinly sliced orange
- Olive oil or melted butter for drizzling

ONE-PAN BAKED ROSEMARY CITRUS SALMON

PREPARATION:

1. Preheat your oven at 400°F / 204°C
2. Whisk orange juice, lemon juice, fresh rosemary, ⅓ cup olive oil, a pinch of salt and pepper, ⅛ of orange peel, and garlic all together and set aside.
3. Next step is to layer your dish, preferably a large deep baking dish, or a roaster.
4. Firstly, add your trimmed asparagus (or your choice of veg) and drizzle with the olive oil (or melted butter). Add a pinch of lemon pepper for seasoning if you like.
5. Skin side down; add your salmon filets on top or in between the asparagus/veg.
6. Drizzle your premade marinade over the fish.
7. Add a layer of orange slices over the fish and the asparagus/veg.
8. Add the 2 sprigs of rosemary on the salmon.
9. Sprinkle some salt, pepper and the left over dried orange peel over the whole pan.
10. Bake for 12 –15 minutes, or until fish is soft and tender in the middle.

VEGETABLE RECIPES

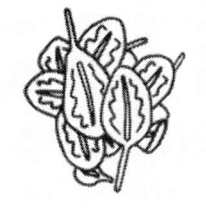

SHEET-PAN ROASTED VEGETABLES

Time: 20 minutes | Serves: 6
Net Carbs: 38.09g | Fiber: 8.6 g | Protein: 4.97 g
Fat: 7.35 g | Kcal (per serving): 221

INGREDIENTS:

- 3 tablespoons olive oil
- 1 tablespoon maple syrup
- 1 tablespoon fresh orange juice
- 2 teaspoons chopped fresh tarragon
- 3 cups butternut squash, peeled and cubed
- 2¼ cups parsnips, peeled and chopped into 1" pieces
- 1lbs of Brussels sprouts, trimmed and halved
- 8oz of small potatoes, halved (Preferably Yukon Gold)
- 1 teaspoon kosher salt
- ½ teaspoon freshly ground black pepper
- 1 teaspoon orange zest strips for seasoning
- 1 tablespoon orange juice for seasoning
- 1 teaspoon chopped fresh tarragon for seasoning
- Cooking spray

PREPARATION:

1. Preheat your oven at 450°F / 232°C.
2. In a bowl, combine the olive oil, maple syrup, orange juice, 2 teaspoons of tarragon, salt and pepper using a whisk.
3. In a large bowl, combine butternut squash, parsnips, Brussels sprouts and potatoes.
4. Add the liquid mixture to the vegetables, and toss to coat everything evenly.
5. Line a baking sheet with some foil and coat with cooking spray.
6. Spread the coated veggies in a single layer onto the baking sheet.
7. Bake for 35 minutes, stirring gently after 25 minutes to ensure even baking.
8. Sprinkle the bake with the seasonings of orange zest strips, orange juice and tarragon.
9. Toss and serve.

BROWN RICE AND PARSLEY PILAF

Time: 40 minutes | Serves: 2
Net Carbs: 40.37 g | Fiber: 2.5 g | Protein: 4.17 g
Fat: 7.42 g | Kcal (per serving): 244

INGREDIENTS:

- ½ cup uncooked brown rice
- 2 teaspoons olive oil
- ⅓ cup chopped yellow onion
- ¼ cup chopped carrot
- 2 teaspoons mince garlic
- 2 tablespoons chopped fresh flat leafed parsley
- 2 teaspoons grated lemon rind
- ½ teaspoon kosher salt
- ¼ teaspoon black pepper

PREPARATION:

1. Using the package directions, cook your rice, but do not add salt or any fats
2. While your rice is cooking, heat olive oil over a medium heat, in a non-stick skillet.
3. Add the onion and the carrot. Cook for about 5 minutes or until tender, stirring occasionally.
4. Add garlic and cook for a further 1 minute.
5. Take off the heat and mix in the parsley, salt and pepper.
6. Put the cooked rice into a large bowl and fluff it with a fork.
7. Add the onion-carrot mixture to the rice and stir to combine.

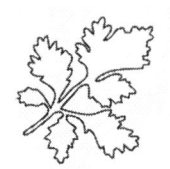

BRAISED FINGERLING POTATOES

Time: 20 minutes | Serves: 3
Net Carbs: 40.37 g | Fiber: 2.5 g | Protein: 4.17 g
Fat: 7.42 g | Kcal (per serving): 244

INGREDIENTS:

- 1 tablespoon olive oil
- 2 teaspoons unsalted butter
- ½ cup white onion, thinly sliced
- 1 lb of fingerling potatoes. Half them length-wise.
- ½ cup of unsalted chicken stock
- 3 sprigs of oregano
- 2 sprigs of thyme
- 1 teaspoon of chopped oregano
- 1 teaspoon of chopped thyme
- ¼ teaspoon of kosher salt
- ¼ teaspoon of black pepper

PREPARATION:

1. Preheat oven to 375°F/190°C
2. In a large, oven-proof skillet, heat olive oil and unsalted butter together, over a medium to high heat.
3. Add the white onion and fingerling potatoes to the skillet, cook for 8 minutes.
4. Add the unsalted chicken stock, oregano and thyme sprigs.
5. Cover the skillet and bake in the over for 10 minutes.
6. Take out the oven and discard the oregano and thyme sprigs.
7. Sprinkle the dish with the chopped oregano, chopped thyme, salt and pepper.

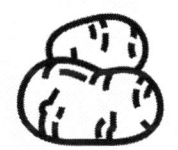

HONEY GLAZED EGGPLANT

Time: 40 minutes | Serves:2
Net Carbs: 80.29 g | Fiber: 17.1 g | Protein: 6.4 g
Fat: 28.61 g | Kcal (per serving): 559

INGREDIENTS:

- 2 large, thinly sliced, eggplants
- ½ teaspoon of salt
- ¼ cup of olive oil
- 5 tablespoons of honey
- 1 juiced large lemon
- 2 minced cloves of garlic
- 2 tablespoons of minced ginger
- 2 teaspoons of cumin
- 1 teaspoon of harissa (or 0.5 teaspoon of hot sauce if harissa is unavailable)
- ½ cup of chopped fresh cilantro
- ½ cup of hot water

PREPARATION:

1. Place your eggplant slices onto a towel and sprinkle all sides with salt. Allow the eggplants to sweat for about 15 minutes and wipe them dry with a paper towel.
2. Preheat a large-sized skillet over a medium high heat.
3. Brush all sides of the eggplants with olive oil and cook until all sides are browned. Try not to crowd the eggplants in the pan, so perhaps do two slices at a time. Remove from pan once done.
4. In a small mixing bowl, combine the honey, lemon juice and hot water until the honey is dissolved.
5. Add the ginger and garlic to the skillet, stir for 30 seconds, and then add the cumin and harissa (or hot sauce).
6. Add the honey mixture to the skillet and stir until boiling.
7. Now add all the eggplant back in the skillet and cook over a medium heat for 10 minutes. After 5 minutes, turn the eggplants to make sure they are fully coated with the sauce.
8. Continue to cook until sauce becomes a thick glaze and eggplant is tender.
9. Garnish with the cilantro (or parsley of you prefer), and serve warm.

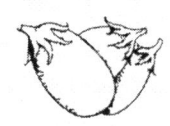

JAMBALAYA VEGAN STYLE

Time: 45 minutes | Serves: 4
Net Carbs: 80.29 g | Fiber: 17.1 g | Protein: 6.4 g
Fat: 28.61 g | Kcal (per serving): 559

INGREDIENTS:

- 1 diced onion
- 2 chopped celery stalks
- 4 minced garlic cloves
- ½ diced green pepper
- ½ diced red pepper
- 14 oz (1can) crushed tomatoes
- 4 cups of vegetable stock
- 1 teaspoon dried oregano
- 1 teaspoon dried basil
- 1 teaspoon dried thyme
- 1 teaspoon of sweet paprika
- ½ teaspoon of smoky paprika
- ½ teaspoon of dried cayenne pepper
- 2 bay leaves
- 2 tablespoons Tabasco sauce (adjust to your taste)
- 2 tablespoons soy sauce
- Salt and pepper to taste
- 2 cups of uncooked brown rice
- 1 cup chickpeas
- 1 cup white beans
- 1 cup kidney beans
- ¼ cup of fresh chopped parsley
- 1 optional green onion

PREPARATION:

1. Over a medium to high heat, heat a large pan and add a tablespoon of oil or water

2. Sauté onion and garlic until tender.

3. Add the celery, peppers and, if necessary, another splash of water. Sauté until just softening.

4. Pour in the crushed tomatoes, vegetable stock, herbs, spices, sauce and rice. Don't add the salt yet! Bring this to a boil, then reduce the heat to allow setting, and cover the pan.

5. Let it simmer for about 30 to 40 minutes, until the rice is cooked and the liquid is all absorbed. Keep stirring now and then to stop the rice from sticking.

6. Once you're happy with the softness of the rice, add the beans and stir. Taste, add salt if necessary.

7. Let it sit on the low heat for about a minute or two to warm the beans and then serve with the parsley (and optional green onion) placed on top.

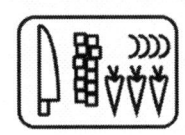

SALAD RECIPES

SALAD RECIPES

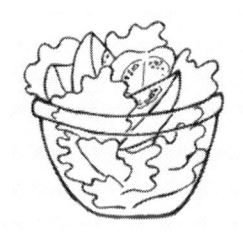

EASY MEDITERRANEAN SALAD

Time: 10 minutes | Serves: 4
Net Carbs: 22.67g | Fiber: 3.6 g | Protein: 4.75g
Fat: 8.99 g | Kcal (per serving): 199

INGREDIENTS:

- 2 cups diced cherry tomatoes
- 1 diced yellow bell pepper
- 1 cup diced red onion
- ½ cup sliced black olives
- 1 sliced medium-sized cucumber
- 3 tablespoons of crumbled feta cheese
- 3 tablespoons julienne cut sun-dried tomatoes
- 3 tablespoons extra virgin olive oil
- 1 teaspoon minced garlic
- 1 tablespoon lemon juice
- 1 teaspoon salt
- 1 teaspoon black pepper
- 1 tablespoon chopped fresh parsley

PREPARATION:

1. Using a large bowl, add the cherry tomatoes, yellow bell pepper, red onions, black olives, cucumber, feta cheese, sun-dried tomatoes and toss together until combined.
2. In a smaller bowl, mix olive oil, garlic, lemon juice, salt and pepper, using a whisk to make the salad dressing.
3. Pour your salad dressing over your salad, and toss to combine.
4. Finish it off with some fresh parsley and serve.

LETTUCE CUPS EGG SALAD

Time: 10 minutes | Serves: 3
Net Carbs: 6.18 g | Fiber: 0.7 g | Protein: 22.15 g
Fat: 20.17 g | Kcal (per serving): 298

INGREDIENTS:

- 5 eggs, hard boiled and peeled
- 1 tablespoon of finely diced red onion
- 1 thinly sliced green onion
- ¼ cup of diced cucumber
- ¼ cup of chopped mixed olives
- ¼ cup of crumbled feta cheese
- 5.3 oz of plain Greek yogurt
- ¼ cup chopped roasted red-peppers
- 1 teaspoon of pepper
- 1 teaspoon of salt
- 6 Romaine lettuce leaves

PREPARATION:

1. Using a large bowl, add the Greek yogurt, cucumber, red onion, green onion, olives, and feta cheese. Mix thoroughly to combine.
2. Slice the eggs; add to the mixture and mix.
3. Taste and add salt and pepper if desired.
4. Add the roasted red-peppers and mix until combined.
5. Use a Romaine lettuce leaf in place of a bowl/plate (ie as an edible plate!) and scoop some salad into it. Continue until all 6 lettuce leaves are filled.

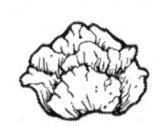

Time: 15 minutes | Serves: 4
Net Carbs: 72.1 g | Fiber: 14.3g | Protein: 25.88 g
Fat: 20.92g | Kcal (per serving): 565

INGREDIENTS:

- 5 oz arugula or your preferred salad greens
- 15oz drained and rinsed chickpeas
- ½ a small-sized red onion
- ½ of a thinly sliced English cucumber
- ½ cup roasted red peppers, diced
- ½ cup feta cheese, crumbled
- 3 tablespoons olive oil
- 1 tablespoon red wine vinegar
- 1 teaspoon Dijon mustard
- 1 teaspoon dried oregano
- ½ teaspoon fine sea salt
- ½ teaspoon freshly cracked black pepper
- 1 small garlic clove, minced (or ½ teaspoon garlic powder)

MEDITERRANEAN SALAD FOR EVERYDAY

PREPARATION:

1. First, let's make the vinaigrette: In a mixing bowl, put the olive oil, red wine vinegar, Dijon mustard, oregano, salt, pepper and minced garlic clove together and whisk until combined.
2. Taste and add a sweetener if you prefer.
3. The vinaigrette can be stored in the fridge for up to 3 days, in a sealed container.
4. In a large salad bowl, toss in all the greens, chickpeas, onion, cucumber, red peppers and feta cheese.
5. Drizzle the vinaigrette evenly over your salad and toss to combine.
6. Serve with some more feta or black pepper if you prefer.

BALELA SALAD

Time: 15 minutes | Serves: 6
Net Carbs: 39.5 g | Fiber: 10 g | Protein: 12.4 g
Fat: 7.6g | Kcal (per serving): 267

INGREDIENTS:

- 3½ cups cooked chickpeas
- ½ chopped green bell-pepper
- 1 optional finely chopped jalapeno
- 2 ½ cups cherry tomatoes
- 3 – 5 green onions, chopped
- ½ cup sun dried tomatoes
- ⅓ cup pitted Kalamate olives
- ¼ cup pitted green olives
- ½ cup chopped fresh parsley
- ½ cup chopped fresh mint leaves
- ¼ cup extra virgin olive oil
- 2 tablespoons white wine vinegar
- 2 tablespoons lemon juice
- 1 minced garlic clove
- Generous pinches salt and pepper
- 1 teaspoon of ground sumac
- ½ teaspoon of Aleppo pepper

BALELA SALAD

PREPARATION:

1. Using a large mixing bowl, mix the chickpeas, vegetables, olives and fresh herbs all together.

2. Using a smaller mixing bowl, add together the dressing Ingredients: namely the olive oil, white wine vinegar, lemon juice, minced garlic, salt, pepper, sumac and Aleppo pepper.

3. Once your dressing is combined, drizzle it over the salad and gently mix to coat everything.

4. Set aside for at least 30 minutes before serving.

5. If you're preparing it long before serving, cover and put in the fridge until ready to serve.

6. Before serving, give the salad a quick stir and a taste. Add some salt if required.

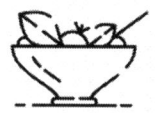

PASTA AND HUMMUS SALAD

Time: 20 minutes | Serves:5
Net Carbs: 27.65 g | Fiber: 4.2 g | Protein: 7.67 g
Fat: 9.66 g | Kcal (per serving): 223

INGREDIENTS:

- 12 oz penne rotini (or any small pasta of your choosing)
- 2 cups broccoli florets
- 1 chopped medium-sized pepper
- 1 chopped onion
- ½ cup kalamata olives
- ¼ cup parmesan cheese
- 2/3 cup hummus
- 1 tablespoon olive oil
- 1 tablespoon water
- 1 teaspoon pepper
- 1 teaspoon of salt
- ½ teaspoon lemon juice

PASTA AND HUMMUS SALAD

PREPARATION:

1. Cook your penne (or your choice of small pasta) according to the package instructions, and let it cool.
2. Using a mixing bowl, add the hummus, water, olive oil, some salt and pepper to taste and stir well to make the salad dressing.
3. In another bowl, add the broccoli, pepper, onion, kalamata olives, cheese, and some salt and pepper and stir to combine.
4. Add the cooled pasta, dressing and mix.

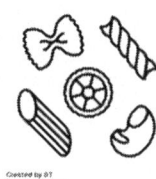

SNACKS & DESSERT RECIPES

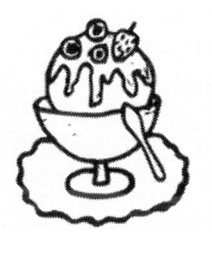

CHOC CHIP COOKIES

Time: 10 minutes | Serves: 24
Net Carbs: 24.97 g | Fiber: 1 g | Protein: 1.7 g
Fat: 6.94g | Kcal (per serving): 170

INGREDIENTS:

- 1 cup extra virgin olive oil
- 1 tablespoon vanilla extract
- ¾ cup granulated sugar
- ¾ cup golden brown sugar
- 1 large egg
- 1 teaspoon Kosher salt (save a bit more for garnishing)
- 2 cups all purpose flour
- ½ teaspoon baking soda
- 2 cups semi-sweet chocolate chips

PREPARATION:

1. Preheat oven to 350°F/180°C
2. Line 2 baking sheets with baking paper/parchment paper.
3. In a large mixing bowl, add olive oil, vanilla, granulated and brown sugars, and salt. Mix until smooth in consistency.
4. Add in the egg and blend until smooth.
5. Add in flour and baking soda. Mix until it is fully combined and there are no dry bits of flour in the mixture.
6. Fold the chocolate chips into the mixture.
7. Using your hands, shape the cookie batter into balls of about 2 tablespoons each.
8. Add the cookie balls to the baking sheets as you go along, keeping them about 2" apart.
9. Gently flatten each ball with your hand palm.
10. Lightly sprinkle each one with the extra salt.
11. Bake the cookies for 10 – 12 minutes, until they are golden brown along the edges.
12. Let cool for about 5 minutes, and then place them on a cooling rack to cool further.

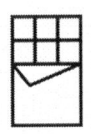

NUTTY CHOC BROWNIES

Time: 10 minutes | Serves: 24
Net Carbs: 12.37 g | Fiber: 1 g | Protein: 3.4 g
Fat: 7.93g | Kcal (per serving): 129

INGREDIENTS:

- ¼ cup extra virgin olive oil
- ¼ cup low fat Greek yogurt
- ¾ cup sugar
- 1 teaspoon vanilla extract
- 2 eggs
- ½ cup of flour
- ⅓ cup of cocoa powder (but you can adjust this as desired)
- ¼ teaspoon of baking powder
- ¼ teaspoon salt
- ⅓ cup of chopped walnuts

PREPARATION:

1. Preheat your oven to 350°F/180°C
2. Line a 9" / 22cm square baking pan with some baking paper.
3. In a mixing bowl, add the olive oil and sugar and mix thoroughly until smooth.
4. Add the vanilla extract and mix well again.
5. Beat eggs in a separate bowl and add to your mixture. Mix well.
6. In another mixing bowl, add the flour, cocoa powder, salt and baking powder and mix well.
7. Add the dry mix to the olive oil mix and mix together well.
8. Add nuts and mix well.
9. Pour the mixture carefully into the lined baking pan and level out the top.
10. Bake for about 25 minutes.
11. Let it completely cool before removing the wax paper and then cut into brownie squares.

CHOC MOUSSE

Time: 2 hours | Serves: 4
Net Carbs: 23.18 g | Fiber: 2.7g | Protein: 17.93 g
Fat: 12.71g | Kcal (per serving): 279

INGREDIENTS:

- ¾ cup of milk
- 3½ oz of dark chocolate
- 1 tablespoon of honey (or you can substitute with maple syrup)
- ½ teaspoon of vanilla extract

PREPARATION:

1. Grate or very finely chop the chocolate.
2. In a saucepan, add the mile and the prepared chocolate.
3. Gently heat the milk until the chocolate has melted, but do not allow it to boil.
4. When the milk and the chocolate have combined, add the honey and vanilla extract and mix together well.
5. In a large mixing bowl, add the Greek yogurt and pour chocolate mixture on top.
6. Mix the chocolate mixture and yogurt together well.
7. Divide the mousse mixture evenly into ramekins or glasses.
8. Place in the fridge to chill for at least 2 hours.
9. Serve with some fresh raspberries and/or a mint leaf.
10. Please note that this mousse, if kept in the fridge, will keep for approximately 2 days.

Time: 15 minutes | Serves:20
Net Carbs: 24 g | Fiber: 3g | Protein: 4 g
Fat: 8g | Kcal (per serving): 170

INGREDIENTS:

- 16 oz semi sweet chocolate
- 1 cup dry quinoa
- 1 tablespoon PB2*
- ½ teaspoon vanilla
- 2 tablespoons water (for the drizzle)
- 2 ½ tablespoons PB2* (for the drizzle)

QUINOA CRUNCHIES

PREPARATION:

1. *PB2 is peanut butter powder and is available online or in health stores.
2. Line a baking sheet with baking paper.
3. First you are going to pop the quinoa. Yes, pop it! Heat a large pot over a medium to high heat for several minutes. Do not add the quinoa yet!
4. Only adding ¼ of the cup at a time add the quinoa to the heated pot. Swirling now and then, let the quinoa sit at the bottom of the cooking pot, until you start hearing a light popping. When it starts popping, swirling continuously until the popping has subsided. Be very careful to not let the quinoa brown, as this can happen very quickly.
5. Once it has all popped, place in a small bowl until required.
6. In a double boiler, melt all your chocolate.
7. In a mixing bowl, add the melted chocolate, popped quinoa, 1 tablespoon of PB2*, and vanilla and mix until combined.
8. Spread the chocolaty-quinoa mixture over the baking sheet. Don't spread too much, as you don't want the crunchies to be too thin. Make it about ½" in thickness.
9. In another mixing bowl, add the 2 tablespoons of water and the 2 ½ tablespoons of PB2* and mix together.
10. Drizzle your drizzle over the top of the chocolaty-quinoa and with a knife, swirl it gently around.
11. Place the baking sheet into the fridge and chill for an hour (minimum!).
12. Slice as desired.

GLAZED PEACHES WITH HAZELNUTS

Time: 30 mins | Serves: 6
Net Carbs: 28.58 g | Fiber: 2.8g | Protein: 2.28 g
Fat: 4.81g | Kcal (per serving): 152

INGREDIENTS:

- 2 tablespoons lemon juice
- 1 tablespoon sugar
- ¼ teaspoon salt
- 6 firm, ripe peaches, peeled, halved, pitted
- ⅓ cup water
- ¼ cup honey
- 1 tablespoon extra virgin olive oil
- ¼ cup hazelnuts. Must be toasted, skinned and chopped coarsely.

GLAZED PEACHES WITH HAZELNUTS

PREPARATION:

1. In your oven, move your rack to 6" from the griller/broiler element.
2. In a large bowl, combine lemon juice, sugar and the salt.
3. Add the peaches and toss to mix together. Ensure the peaches are coasted evenly on all sides.
4. In a 12" oven safe skillet, arrange the coated peach halves and pour any remaining sugary syrup onto them.
5. Pour water into the skillet, around the peaches.
6. Grill the peaches until they are just beginning to brown, around 11 to 15 minutes.
7. In a bowl, add the honey and oil together and warm in the microwave for about 20 seconds. Stir to mix together.
8. Remove the skillet from the grill and brush HALF of the honey onto the peaches.
9. Replace under the grill for another 5 to 7 minutes, until they are spotty brown.
10. Take out the oven and brush with the remaining honey.
11. Place peaches on a serving platter.
12. There should be some peach juice left in the skillet. Place this on a medium heat, let simmer. Whisk frequently to combine for 1 minute or until it turns syrupy.
13. Pour this over the peaches and cover them with the hazelnuts.

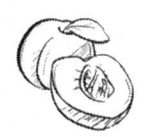

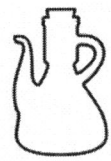

As we have mentioned throughout, the Mediterranean diet seems to offer one of the best meal plans there is when it comes to staying in shape and losing weight. Apart from a lot of walking that people living in villages of this region do daily, it is the diet that keeps them healthy and slim. Oh yes, and low-stress life in general. But is this not a bit contradictory, bearing in mind that we are talking about meals and foods that are quite high in fat? Well, not at all. The thing is, you will be eating the *right* type of fat. Now, we don't want to say that saturated fat is going to kill you, but it should be eaten in moderation, unless you want to feel the ill effects of it relating weight and cardiovascular health. Saturated fat is present in meats, eggs and other products that are common for the diet. On the other hand, a typical Mediterranean plate would include close to non-meat products, as fish, whole grains, and vegetables are the core of this diet. But is the lack of meat and saturated fat all there is to it when it comes to losing weight? No, but it certainly helps.

There are a number of benefits connected to meals that are typical for this region. As many studies suggest, patients that have been eating the Mediterranean diet for a longer time, have a significantly less chance of developing a cardiovascular disease. In fact, from what it seems, eating a diet rich in omega 3 and omega 6 fats, as well as whole grains, minerals and vitamins, will work like a charm when it comes to your overall health. Following this concept will result in you having lower levels of LDL while maintaining higher levels of HDL (high-density lipoprotein cholesterol) as well as steady blood pressure. Further benefits include higher levels of energy, as well as better memory and focus. Additionally, following such a meal plan will pump your body with antioxidants (here red wine plays quite a role) that are critical for fighting off free radicals and reducing chances of cancer. So with all these benefits in mind, surely it is better to get up and cook yourself a tasty and colorful meal, instead of going to visit a fast food chain? But if you are having trouble with weight, and finding it difficult to lose those few pounds, what kind of a meal plan should you follow and what are the tips that will allow you optimal results? Let's go ahead and take a look at the few that we have prepared for you!

Eat Your Main Meal Early

We are not saying that you should eat your lunch before breakfast, but we are suggesting that instead of eating your main meal at 4-5 PM, it would be much better if you did so before 3 PM. This is something that is pretty common for people in the Mediterranean region, and there is a good reason for it. If you eat a large meal earlier in the day, chances are you will eat less later on. It is a common habit that allows, for example, Italians to eat more than one plate of food for lunch while staying in great shape!

Vegetables and Olive Oil – The Perfect Combination

Apart from eating these in a salad, one of the good things you can do is to eat a few servings of vegetables by cooking them in olive oil. This is a tastier and more efficient way of getting your micronutrients. There are a number of vegetables that end up being even better once you cook them including zucchini, eggplant, carrots, and tomatoes (though they are technically a fruit). Pair this with some feta cheese and you will enjoy a wonderful meal!

Hydrate, Hydrate, Hydrate

Much like with any other diet, it is critical to drink good amounts of water throughout the whole day. Water is the key to life and without it, we would not be able to function properly. Drinking at least 8 glasses of H2O will better your digestive system and allow you to stay energized. Other than water, wine is a common drink of choice for adults. You can enjoy this as well, as long as you are not going over 1-2 glasses, at most, a day. The main reason the Mediterranean diet includes wine, is due to its abundance of antioxidants. Coffee and tea are perfectly fine as well, and may even contribute to boosting your metabolism.

Don't Run Away From Olive Oil

Yes, oil is fats and fats have a greater caloric-density than proteins or carbs, which means they keep you full for a longer time. The main thing about olive oil is that it is rich and has a great balance of omega 3 and omega 6 fatty acids which are vital for your cardiovascular and brain health. Also, no one can deny that olive oil is quite tasty and it is great for cooking as well. A few tablespoons of olive oil a day will work like a charm.

Walk This Day

The importance of regular exercise is huge when it comes to losing weight, and following the Mediterranean diet. Taking a light walk, or doing some gardening after your meal, will be a great way to get your exercise in without overwhelming yourself. Other than that, be sure to engage in some kind of sports or workout regime a few times a week. Don't forget that sleep is equally as important, so try to get anywhere from 6-8 hours a night.

Eat Right

This one is quite clear. Eating the right foods will be of immense help when it comes to losing weight over a short period of time. A Mediterranean diet consists of a lot of vegetables, whole grains, nuts, fruits, fish, and low-fat dairy products. Making these a part of your every meal, whether it be a soup, yogurt dessert, a nice masala, or a pasta dish, will let you get the much-needed micro and macronutrients and be on your way to achieving optimum weight-loss results.

Avoid The Wrong Foods

As much as eating right is important, it is probably even more to avoid the wrong foods and ingredients. What you shouldn't eat is mostly refined products including processed sugars, trans fats, and meat such as sausages and hot dogs. Also, you should skip on eating in fast food chains and restaurants, but instead, enjoy spending time in the kitchen experimenting with tasty and versatile recipes.

Stay Strict

If you don't follow your regime and schedule, you won't get great results. If you want to lose a lot of weight in a short period of time, following the Mediterranean diet you shouldn't think about cheat meals and days. The reason? Food in this meal plan is already tasty and exotic enough, that once you prepare it the right way, there is no need to alter anything.

Enjoy Your Food

A common habit for people in the Mediterranean region is that they eat together and savor each and every bite. That is what you should indulge in, as well as the whole atmosphere related to this concept, will allow you break from the day and actually stay in the moment.

Festina Lente

Last but not least is, as the Ancient Romans used to say, you should simply slow down and take things with less stress. People tend to go rushing here and everywhere and don't pay enough respect to food or themselves. Believe it or not, this is also a trigger for obesity, as high levels of cortisol lead to weight gain.

Doing research on the Mediterranean diet and common recipes was an enjoyable task and something that should prove of great value to all of us. We truly hope that this cookbook will be of great help to you, whether you simply want to understand more about the region and their food habits, lose weight or improve cooking skills. Among all other things and benefits that come with this concept, we do see one as the most crucial, and that is to take a break and enjoy our food, drinks, and life. With this attitude and the Mediterranean diet, only sky will be the limit to what you can achieve!

DISCLAIMER

DISCLAIMER

The opinions and ideas of the author contained in this publication are designed to educate the reader in an informative and helpful manner. While we accept that the instructions will not suit every reader, it is only to be expected that the recipes might not gel with everyone. Use the book responsibly and at your own risk. This work with all its contents, does not guarantee correctness, completion, quality or correctness of the provided information. Always check with your medical practitioner should you be unsure whether to follow a low carb eating plan. Misinformation or misprints cannot be completely eliminated. Human error is real!

Cover: oliviaprodesign
Cover Photo: somegirl / depositphotos.com

Printed by Amazon Italia Logistica S.r.l.
Torrazza Piemonte (TO), Italy